A Salute to America's #1 N

MUSCADINE Power

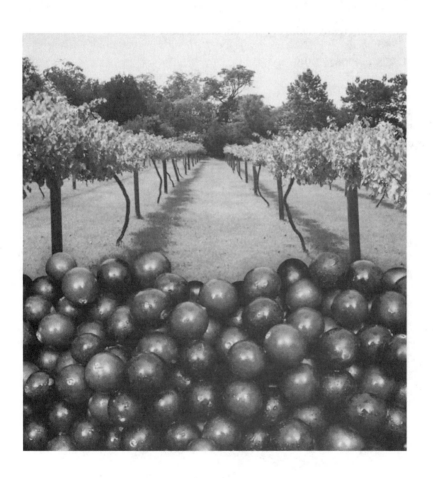

Dr. Allan C. Somersall, PhD, MD

Copyright © 2008/2014

Library of Congress Cataloging-in-Publication Data

ISBN 978-0-9906177-0-9

Printed in USA
First Edition, June 2008
Second Edition, July 2014

10 9 8 7 6

This report is intended for educational purposes only and makes no claims to diagnose or treat any disease or condition.

Statements herein have **not** been evaluated by the US Food and Drug Administration.

Contents

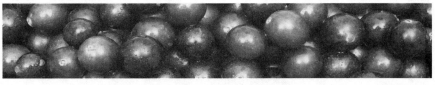

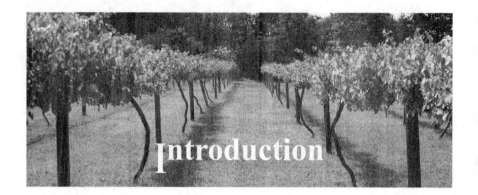

Introduction

Who would have guessed 400 years ago, when Native Americans bit into those big, luscious berries growing wild in wood margins or hedgerows of the southeastern United States, that they were fortifying their bodies with phytochemicals that would later prove to be among the most protective health foods found anywhere on the planet.

It was no accident of history that the health benefits to be derived from those same muscadine grapes that the Native Americans came to treasure, have now been proven scientifically to be vital and even more relevant to Americans in the 21st Century, when chronic degenerative diseases have become the major killers.

These were no ordinary grapes. Muscadines are in a class all by themselves. Right at the core of their DNA, they have been programmed for distinction. **An extra pair of chromosomes endowed muscadine berries (which they technically are) with a unique combination of phytochemicals** that first protected them from *their* environmental challenges and hazards. But what was originally designed to benefit the plant and its produce, turns out to be also very beneficial to the human body. When consumed, as we shall see, some of these same natural products from the grapevine also conferred nutraceutical and even true medicinal benefits to humans.[1]

People around the country are now using muscadine products to help protect their heart, improve cholesterol profiles, control blood sugar, reduce cancer risk, fight inflammation, help erectile dysfunction, and even look and feel younger.

As you go through this booklet, you will learn much more about the nutritional and nutraceutical ingredients of muscadines and the important roles they play in both health and disease. You will learn about the new approaches to the science of nutrition. It focuses far less today on the well-known *macro*nutrients that are principally sources of energy and body mass (like proteins, carbohydrates and fats), and even less on the traditional *micro*nutrients that control metabolism and repair body tissues (like vitamins and minerals). Rather, you will be introduced to a new world of cell protectors - mainly antioxidants and free radical scavengers. These amazing bioactive, protective molecules that are not yet familiar to the public at large, have been provided in nature for thousands of years. But only in the past few decades have scientists begun to understand their critical value in health and disease. That's because we have now come to realize the central role that **free radicals** themselves play in disease processes.

It seems like free radicals are showing up everywhere. Where do they come from? We now appreciate that a range of different processes give rise to highly reactive molecules with unpaired electrons, inside cells and on cellular surfaces. You could be exposed to these harmful free radicals by any of the sources on the following short list:

- Both normal and abnormal *metabolic processes* taking place in the body can create free-radical intermediates.

- In the course of industrial processing of foods with the inclusion of synthetic *food additives*, free radicals are introduced. These are being increasingly consumed every day.

- There is often exposure to *chemical contaminants* in the environment - including air and water, both in the home and in the workplace.

- Primary *pollutants from smoking* include free radicals. So do the consequences and side effects of secondhand smoke.

- Biochemical intermediates in the body can be due to the metabolism and detoxification of some *medications.*

Oxygen is the most vital input into the body. There is no life without it. However, free radicals react readily with oxygen to cause premature oxidation of cells and tissues. This wreaks havoc in the body. The unstable and aggressive intermediates can attack DNA, leading to all kinds of cellular mutation and disease. *Antioxidants* are molecules that help the body to protect itself from the damage and rigors of such premature oxidation. Nature provides thousands of examples of antioxidants. Some are intrinsic to normal cellular activity or otherwise enhanced from dietary sources. Intrinsic to the cells for example, would be the tripeptide called *glutathione,* which is considered by many to be the master intracellular antioxidant. Dietary antioxidants, on the other hand, would include the well known vitamins C and E, and the trace mineral, selenium.

The research in the past few decades has already indicated that the best sources of natural antioxidants are fruits and vegetables. Among these, **the most powerful antioxidants turn out to be some of the phytonutrients found particularly in the mighty muscadines and other dark-skinned berries**. And that's not all. Some phenolic compounds in muscadines (again, we will see later), like resveratrol, ellagic acid and quercetin, (just to name a few), produce specific responses such as reducing inflammation and improving the health of the heart and other organs.

To illustrate how important these findings about muscadines could be, just consider the following list of diseases that the experts are actively studying with respect to the effects of antioxidants and anti-inflammatory agents:

Allergies	Immune suppression	Hypertenstion
Rheumatoid Arthritis	Osteoporosis	Heart disease
Cancer	Parkinson's disease	Schizophrenia
Diabetes	DNA mutations	Atheroscelerosis
Gum disease	Birth defects	Cataracts
Crohn's disease	Alzheimer's disease	... etc., etc.

That's also a short list, but central to many of these conditions, is the ability to regulate gene expression. Surprising as it may seem, phytonutrients in the muscadine grapes are now known to affect gene expression and processes as fundamental as cell growth and replication.

You've probably heard of other foods in the media with a popular reputation for healthy ingredients. Those might include blueberries, goji berries, green tea, acai grapes, noni juice, red wine and even dark chocolate. Add to that abbreviated list, perhaps garlic, broccoli, cayenne pepper, ginger, spinach, tomatoes ... and the list could go on. But at the top of the 'healthy foods' pyramid, with nutraceuticals *par excellence*, **eventually you will find the muscadine grape that surpasses them all. It has a myriad of biochemically active ingredients that now threaten to spawn another** *nutritional revolution.*

There's a lot to learn about muscadines, but before we go deep into this exciting area of scientific interest and consumer curiosity, we should back up and find out where this all began. And it started right here in the United States.

2. A Brief History of Muscadines [2.]

Muscadine grapes are indeed native to the southeastern United States where they have been cultivated for a few hundred years. Long before the first Europeans arrived on this side of the Atlantic, the Native Americans had already discovered the value of this grapevine species which was growing wild on the coastal plains of North and South Carolina, Virginia, Georgia, and their neighboring states. They had already begun to enjoy unintentional health benefits by eating the whole ripe berries themselves, drinking their juice and preserving them as dried fruit and raisins for later treats. They were standard fare. They created traditional recipes, some of which are still popular today, including 'Cherokee dumplings'. The grapes were sometimes referred to then as '*possum grapes*'.

The earliest record of the occurrence of muscadine grapevines was documented back in 1524 by the navigator Giovanni de Verrazzano. He was from Florence, Italy and was hired as a ship captain by the French king to explore and report on the habitat of the New World and its inhabitants, 30 years after Christopher Columbus first set foot here. Captain Verrazzano described a big 'white grape' (later to become known as a *scuppernong* variety of muscadine) that he found growing in great profusion at a valley in Cape Fear, North Carolina.

He wrote of the Native Americans' esteem for these grapes: "*They must be held in estimation by them, as they carefully remove the shrubbery from around them, wherever they grow, to allow the fruit to ripen better.*" Respect for muscadines did go back that far, even though research obviously did not. Sometimes consumers do lead the way.

Another Captain, John Hawkins, also described the Indians' love for muscadines in his sailing records of 1585. He reported that Spanish settlements in Florida made large quantities of muscadine wine. The early varieties were not exotic, but simple selections from the wild. They did not quite get it right, but at least they got it. They did find that *'a little wine was good for* much more than *the stomach's sake.'*

There's a letter written to the English explorer Sir Walter Raleigh in 1584, and ascribed to Arthur Barlowe, an early settler who seemed obviously overwhelmed by what he found in North Carolina, and described the fruitful land as being "*so full of grapes, as the very beating and surge of the sea overflowed them ... that I think in all the world, the like abundance is not to be found.*" They were "*on the sand and on the green soil, on the hills as on the plains, as well as on every little shrub ... also climbing towards the tops of tall cedars ...*" He was clearly impressed by the sheer *quantity* of his discovery, but later generations of colonists and true-blue Americans in the South were to be invigorated by the superior *quality* of this rich-fruit delicacy.

Sir Walter responded to that letter the following year when he himself observed the mother-vine of the scuppernong muscadine on Roanoke Island. It had '*a base thickness of the grape vine stalk of two feet through. The huge vine covered half an acre, coiling up tree trunks growing 60 feet tall.*' Grapes were harvested in large numbers and supplied the mother vineyard winery with fruit to be fermented into 'Virginia Dove' wine in Mantes, NC. This famous wine was pink, aromatic and comparable to port wine. It was destined to become after World War I, at least for some time, the best selling if not best loved wine in America.

The first recognized (named) muscadine cultivar (variety) was a bronze selection, found before 1760 by Isaac Alexander in Tywell County, NC. He was one of two hunters who had to penetrate some dense thickets surrounding a local vine. That day, the plant and the fruits they found surpassed whatever animal game they may have caught. It was first known as the 'Big White Grape' and was later labeled as the *scuppernong* variety referred to earlier, so named after the area in which it was found - along the banks of a short stream, which was called Scuppernong Lake. But it should also be noted that during the 17th and 18th centuries, cuttings of the 'Big White Crops' were placed by the settlers around a small town called Scuppernong in Washington County, NC.

The North Carolina Wine and Grape Council reports that : "*James Blount of the town of Scuppernong took the census of Washington County, NC in 1810 and reported 1,368 gallons of wine made there. A report in the Star newspaper by Dr. Calvin Jones, dated January 11, 1811 commented on Blout's report and that was the first written record of the grape being referred to as a 'scuppernong grape'. Eight years later in 1819, Nathaniel Macon, a member of Congress, sent samples of scuppernong wine to President Thomas Jefferson.*"

It has also been reported that President Jefferson later planted vineyards and harvested muscadines at his home at Monticello. He is also credited with establishing the fruit gardens at the White House in Washington DC in the early 1800's.

As time passed, the scuppernong name became synonymous with all *white* to *bronze* muscadines (and sometimes, all the muscadines), regardless of the actual variety. But in fact, scuppernong is only one of the many cultivars of muscadine grapes. The other general category apart from the bronze grapes ('white' muscadines), would be the purple or black varieties - sometimes called the 'red' muscadines.

North Carolina takes great pride in its muscadine heritage and has proclaimed the muscadine grape as its state fruit as of 2001. This state is considered to be the home of America's first cultivated 'white grape'.

However, North Carolina does not have an exclusive claim on muscadine. In fact, muscadine grapes are found in the wild - from Delaware down to the Gulf of Mexico, and as far west as Missouri, Kansas, Oklahoma and Texas. Commercial production of muscadine grapes is essentially limited to the US southeast. That's mainly because of the grapevine requirements.

3. The Muscadine Grapevine

Muscadines are well adapted to the warm, humid conditions of the southeastern US, where the normal American supermarket grapes and European grapes do not prosper. This empowered species of grapes thrives on summer heat, and lacks any frost hardiness. That limits the muscadine grapevines to this region, with the possible exception of some West Coast locations. They can be grown in California and adjacent areas, but they do not adapt well as other cultivated grapes. In some areas of the West, the lack of sufficient summer heat produces berries that tend to be small and generally low in sugar, whereas in many interior sections, the vines do not fare well in the low humidity. The vines that do make it in the few growing regions of California, Oregon and the state of Washington, produce muscadines that just don't have the same hardiness or deliver the same bounty of phytochemicals.

The species of muscadines is technically known as *Vitis rotundifolia*, because *vitis* is the old Latin name for 'grape' and *rotundifolia* refers to the roundish leaves. These grapes must clearly be distinguished from their less erudite cousins:

- *Vitis vinifera*, the European grapevine native to the Mediterranean and Central Asia.

- *Vitis labrusca*, the North American grapevines that produce table juice, sometimes used for wine. They are Native to the Eastern US and Canada.

- *Vitis riparia*, a wild vine of North America, sometimes used for winemaking and for jam. They are native to the entire Eastern US and further north to Quebec.

- *Vitis vulpine*, a frost grape native to the US Midwest and east to the coast, up through New York.

- *Vitis amurensis*, the most important Asian Species.

There is also a sea grape, *Coccolaba uvifera*, which is actually a member of a different family called *Polygonaceae*, and is native to the Caribbean islands.

So, what's all this fuss about muscadines in the *vitis* family? Is there something really special about this robust grapevine species. YES, there surely is!! Muscadines have 40 chromosomes in their DNA, unlike all the other grape cousins which only have 38. This is no accident of nature and is not without consequences.

We now know that chromosomes contain the genes that provide the blueprint for all the living cell enzymes and proteins. It is therefore not surprising that the **extra pair of chromosomes** in the muscadines give them additional genetic information that really packs a mighty punch.

- **That's why** muscadines can survive the high heat and humidity of the southeastern US.

- **That's why** they grow best in fertile sandy loam and alluvial soils, or why they can grow wild in well-drained bottom lands that are not subject to extended drought or waterlogging.

- **That's why** they are also resistant to pests and diseases, including Pierce's disease, which can wipe out similar species of grapes.

- **That's why** muscadine is one of the grape species most resistant to *Phylloxera*, an insect that can kill off the roots of grapevines.

- **That's why** muscadine grapes have a thicker skin to protect these valuable berries from the devastation caused by heat, ultraviolet radiation, humidity, insects and fungi.

We really don't know which specific genes are on the extra pair of chromosomes found in the muscadines, but they must certainly allow this amazingly resilient gift of nature to develop its own unique balance of phytochemicals, some of which are virtually absent in other grapes.

And here's the really good news. What nature conveniently developed as '*adaptogenic phytochemicals*' to help the muscadine survive and really thrive in challenging environmental conditions, just happens to be of great nutritional and even medicinal value to *homo sapiens,* when we have the pleasure of consuming them. What makes 'the mighty muscadine' show all the characteristics of 'the smarter grape,' turns out in fact to be the best kept health secret in America.' It turns out to be the healthiest grape of all - the richest nutraceutical food known on the planet!

This Is The All-American Grape!

Muscadines are vigorous, deciduous vines that typically grow some 60-100 feet in the wild. They have a tight, non-shedding bark, with warty shoots and unbranched tendrils. The slightly lobed leaves measure 2.5-5 inches and are rounded or broadly ovate, with coarsely serrated edges and an acuminate point. These leaves are dark green above and a green tinged yellow below. They are glossy on both sides and become more firm with maturity. The small, greenish muscadine flowers are borne in short, dense panicles and pollination is facilitated by both wind and insects.

Muscadines have 40 chromosomes in their DNA, unlike all the other grape cousins which only have 38.

But what's the value of a vine if it bore no fruit? What if it had 'nothing but leaves'?

4. The Muscadine Grape

However, the fruit of the muscadines is where the action is. This is a healthy vine that '*bringeth forth fruit ... much fruit ... and even more fruit.*'

Whereas European and American grapes grow in tight, characteristic bunches, the muscadines bear small, loose clusters of 3-40 grapes. The grapes are round, about 1-1.5 inches in diameter and 5-15 grams in weight. They have a thick, tough skin that locks in the essential goodness. The pulp inside surrounds up to five hard, oblong seeds which we will soon learn, have the highest nutritional content of all. Yet at least in quantity, the berries are about 50% pulp, 40% skin and 10% seed. But don't be deceived.

The fruits range in color from a greenish bronze, through bronze, purplish red and purple, to almost black. The content of phytochemicals varies across that spectrum.

Unlike other grapes that grow and mature in tight bunches, the ripe muscadine fruits drop individually from the loose clusters as they ripen. A common harvesting method is simply to spread a sheet or tarpaulin underneath the vine, and then give the stalk a good shake. The grapes start ripening in mid September to late October and in good conditions, a mature vine can yield up to 20 pounds or more of the coveted fruit.

Muscadine grapes are pleasant enough to eat out of hand, despite the seeds and somewhat tough skin. The children in the southeast learn to bite through the skin to get at the pulp and juice which tends to be sweet and somewhat aromatic. The locals boast that **one experience of this pure delight and every other grape would become a disappointment.**

But again, there's more to good food than a sweet taste. The real value is in the skin and seeds which have been regrettably discarded much too often. By the time you finish this monograph, you certainly won't make such an unhealthy mistake. You'll be anxious to benefit from all the nutraceutical value of rich muscadines, in one form or another. There will be different products to choose from.

5. Muscadine Products

Muscadines are now grown commercially across the southeastern US, in hundreds of small vineyards that constitute an industry which has grown considerably over the past 40 years. Today, muscadine products of one type or another have become available throughout the year in markets around the world.

In the late summer or early fall, visitors to the region could be treated to *fresh berries*. These big, beautiful and luscious fruits are sold in super-markets, growers' stands, and the popular, local farmers' markets. You can choose from the bronze or purple varieties, known locally as the *whites* or *reds*. Either cultivar of good quality will deliver a phenomenal treat. That's a highlight of any holiday in the area.

Fresh berries are not available all year round. But different parts of the fruit can be preserved for continuous distribution. The seeds or skins are dried and powdered to produce encapsulated products. With the small par-ticle size, and therefore large surface area, this is a very convenient form for digestion and phytochemical absorption.

Seeds and skins can also be extracted into different oils and solvents to afford choice fractions of different nutraceutical ingredients. As expected, seed *extracts* do not wholly contain the high fiber content of the pulverized seeds.

Muscadine *skins and seeds* are now highly prized sources of phytonutri-ents for use in the food supplement and nutraceutical industries. **Up to 90% of the medicinal value of the muscadine grape resides in the skin and seed fractions,** which until very recently, was discarded as unneces-sary waste residue. That was when muscadine grapes were considered first as fruits for making wines and preserves. But with increased knowl-edge of the powerful antioxidants and much, much more that nature has provided in the muscadine package, each fraction is now considered to be of the highest nutraceutical value. In the dry and powdered forms, in par-ticular, the phytochemicals in the skins and seeds are much more concen-trated than in the whole fruit, and they possess a much longer shelf life for convenient distribution and use. In addition, these powders retain the fiber content and the completely balanced nutrient repertoire that nature has provided in the muscadine *piéce de résistance.*

All year round and right across the nation and beyond, the good taste and nutritious bounty of muscadine fruits are available in an assortment of products like jellies, jams, preserves, pies, sauces, purees and ciders. Hundreds of wholesalers, retailers and mail order suppliers are enjoying a brisk business catering to the demand of initiated consumers. But '*all that glitters is not gold*' and '*you should not judge a book by its cover.*' Muscadine products (forget the implied associations) may almost invariably come short of the new standard of nutraceutical product authenticity. The best you can do is probably to use a concentrated supplement of muscadines from the best available sources.

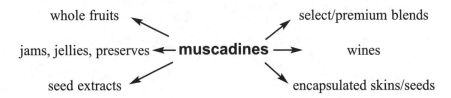

Most muscadines grown commercially are juiced. The juice is either bottled as a 100% unadulterated product or it is mixed with other nutritional components to make *select or premium blends.* One could hardly think of a more delicious or more nutritious, non-alcoholic, beverage alternative to serve the best of company or most distinguished guests at any time. By the way, if settlings ever appear in a bottle of juice, remember that those precipitates represent the highest nutritional content. So, don't forget to shake well before serving.

Muscadine *wines* of both red and white varieties, are now being shipped all over the world. Fermentation of the grapes is not unlike the usual process in wineries. However, the presence of phytonutrients in these wines in particular, adds additional health benefits, as we will soon see.

Health benefits? Aren't muscadines just mere grapes, after all? Yes and No - they are grapes for sure, but a different species indeed. Let's find out.

6. The Nutritional Profile of Muscadines

Although the muscadine grape represents a real powerhouse of phytonu-trients that are invaluable to health, it is still formally classified as a 'food'. Of course it is. It grows naturally on a vine and the luscious berries appeal to you like any other fruit. As such it takes its rightful place among the important dietary category of 'fruits and vegetables.'

Speaking of fruits and vegetables, this brings us to the new US Department of Agriculture Food Guide Pyramid issued in 2005. The recommendations in the ***USDA Dietary Guidelines for Americans*** [3.] are for the general pub-lic over two years of age, and they describe a healthy diet as one that:

- *"Emphasizes fruits, vegetables and whole grains, and fat-free or low-fat milk and milk products;*

- *Includes lean meats, poultry, fish, beans, eggs, and nuts; and*

- *Is low in saturated fats, trans fats, cholesterol, salt (sodium) and added sugars. "*

That's the official word as it appears on the government websites, and you must notice the very first phrase in that specific summary. It '*emphasizes fruits*...' That's more than coincidence, even if it were not intentional. Any ideal dietary guidelines deserve to begin that way. Fruits *can* and per-haps even *should* take center stage.

In the USDA guidelines, the diet is represented as a rainbow of colors arranged in a pyramid (or series of pyramids, to be more precise). There is no doubt that fruits figure prominently in the panorama of foods which are largely 'whole' foods. And yes, they should be. Berries also stand out among the various fruits identified as 'commonly' eaten fruits - which include *"strawberries, blueberries, raspberries and cherries."* Whole grapes are prominently displayed, and the guidelines also include raisins, which are dried grapes. But the **muscadines are most conspicuous by their absence** from the explicit list. That's because these precious grapes are still today, America's best kept health secret.

Further, *"any fruit or 100% fruit juice counts as part of the 'fruit group'. Such fruits may be fresh, canned, frozen or dried, and may be whole, cut-up, or pureed."* This is in contrast to the ever popular all-American soft drinks - carbonated and non-carbonated - representing a drain of billions of hard earned dollars. Yet they provide essentially only water, sugar (empty calories galore), flavor, and carbon dioxide gas. Fruit 'drinks' are not much better. These counterfeits are commercialized formulations which may or may not actually contain natural fruit juice or concentrate. They are often loaded with high-fructose corn syrup sweeteners and food additives to improve palatability, flavor, color, and shelf life. They are designed more for the consumers' convenience and pleasure, and perhaps just as much for the manufacturers' and distributors' profits.

> These precious grapes are still today, America's best kept health secret.

Fruit and fruit juices, on the other hand, do contribute significantly to the nutrient intake of any healthy diet. Consider the observations from the *USDA Dietary Guidelines* again:

- *"Most fruits are naturally low in fat, sodium and calories - None have cholesterol (which is always animal-derived).*

- *Fruits are important sources of many nutrients, including potassium, dietary fiber, vitamin C and folate (folic acid).*

- *Diets rich in potassium may help to maintain healthy blood pressure. Fruit sources of potassium include bananas, prunes (dried plums) and prune juice, dried peaches and apricots, cantaloupe, honeydew melon, and orange juice.*

17

- *Dietary fiber from fruits, as part of an overall healthy diet, helps reduce blood cholesterol levels and may lower risk of heart disease. Fiber is important for proper bowel function. It helps reduce constipation and diverticulosis. Fiber-containing foods, such as fruits, help provide a feeling of fullness with fewer calories - whole or cut-up fruits are sources of dietary fiber; fruit pieces contain little or no fiber.*

- *Vitamin C is important for growth and repair of all body tissues, helps heal cuts and wounds and keeps teeth and gums healthy.*

- *Folate (folic acid) helps the body form red blood cells. Women of child bearing age who may become pregnant and those in the first trimester of pregnancy should consume adequate folate, including folic acid from fortified foods or supplements. This reduces the risk of neural tube defects, spina bifida and anencephaly during fetal development."*

The USDA got it right, but again, with the notable exception of not including muscadine by name. That's not bias, and it's clearly not deliberate. All the nutritional facts about muscadines could propel it into the guidelines for sure. But the American public remains unaware to date. Hopefully, that's not for very much longer. The muscadine secret is out!

Muscadines are low in fat, with moderate levels of protein and carbohydrate. This carbohydrate includes a balance of fructose, glucose and sucrose. Importantly, fructose (the 'fruit sugar') does not raise blood glucose, and this is nature's balance, after all. Muscadines also have very little sodium and yet a healthy amount of potassium. **They are an excellent source of fiber, as much as 50% higher than cooked oatmeal,** which the media would have you believe is the standard for a cholesterol-busting food. According to the FDA, a food that has at least 0.6 gm of soluble fiber per serving without fortification (and muscadine certainly does) can make the following claim: *low fat diets rich in fiber may reduce the risk of some types of cancer, and may reduce the risk of heart disease.* The full nutrient deck for muscadine grapes is given in **Table 1.**

Table 1. Essential nutrients in 100g (3.5 oz.) serving of Muscadine

Nutrient	Bronze-skinned	Dark-skinned
Calories	68	76
Protein	0.5g	0.5g
Fat	0.4g	0.4g
Carbohydrates	12g	14g
Sodium	5mg	7mg
Calcium	17mg	24mg
Potassium	163mg	167mg
Magnesium	5mg	5mg
Vitamin C	7mg	6mg
Dietary Fiber	3mg	3mg
Soluble Fiber	1g	1g

* Compiled by Dr. Betty J. Ector, Mississippi State Nutritionist [4.]

But it is of interest to note that the new *USDA Dietary Guidelines* did not stop there. With the ever increasing understanding of the intricate relationship between diet and health, those guidelines were obliged to identify the health benefits associated with each food category. They were most explicit in concluding that eating fruits provides health benefits - *"peoplewhoeat more fruits and vegetables as part of an overall healthy diet are likely to have reduced risk of some chronic diseases."* Fruits provide nutrients vital for health and maintenance of your body. They go on to be more particular:

- *"Eating a diet rich in fruits and vegetables as part of an overall healthy diet may reduce risk for* **stroke** *and perhaps other* **cardiovascular disease.**

- *Eating a diet rich in fruits and vegetables as part of an overall diet may reduce risk for* **type 2 diabetes.**

- *Eating a diet rich in fruits and vegetables as part of an overall diet may protect against* **cancers,** *such as mouth, stomach, and colon-rectum cancer.*

- *Diets rich in foods containing fiber, such as fruits and vegetables, may reduce the risk of **coronary heart disease.***

- *Eating fruits and vegetables rich in potassium as part of an overall healthy diet may reduce the risk of developing **kidney stones** and may help to decrease **bone loss.***

- *Eating foods such as fruits that are low in calories per cup instead of some other higher-calorie food may be useful in helping to lower calorie intake."* Especially at a time when (a) the US Surgeon General has issued clear warnings about the increasing obesity epidemic in America, and (b) a high restriction in calorie intake (reduced by about one-third) has proven to be consistent with anti-aging effects in laboratory animals.

We have come a long way baby! A few decades ago, we thought of foods so differently. In fact, vitamins were only discovered at the beginning of the last century. It has taken another hundred years to begin to figure out what else nature has always provided in foods for the service of man. And we have only just begun. We still have a long way to go.

The cutting edge of research today is no longer in the traditional nutrient classes: amino acids and proteins; carbohydrate and fiber; fats and free fatty acids, vitamins and minerals. That includes a total list of less than 50 individual dietary ingredients altogether. However, we have neglected the other hundreds of food ingredients that nature intended to provide health and protection to the animal kingdom, especially man.

That brings us to the vast, intimidating but exciting new area of phytochemicals and phytochemical research. There, muscadines will have an even more prominent role.

7. The Phytochemical Content of Muscadine

We've used the term *'phytochemical'* several times already. It's a daunting word and just the reference to anything *'chemical'* sometimes is very misleading. All matter is essentially composed of chemicals - made up of 'molecules' - if you like. Therefore *'chemical'* does not imply synthetic or man-made. It can be all-natural. The prefix *'phyto'* is from the Greek *'phyton,'* meaning plant. So, **phytochemicals are nothing more than chemicals manufactured in plants** - all natural and all of biological significance. They exist in balance and in harmony with nature.

Phytochemicals have assumed a new importance in the biomedical sciences in general, because research is proving every day that Hippocrates did have a meaningful case when he suggested: *'Let food be your medicine and medicine your food.'* He foresaw that ... way back in 400 BC. Today the injunction has new meaning, especially when muscadines are considered.

In addition to the exceptional nutrient profile we described for the muscadine grape, there are at least one hundred other important chemicals, some of which have been isolated, identified and characterized by chemists who specialize in Natural Products. That is a sub-specialty of chemistry, all its own. They are very interesting molecules but unfortunately for the lay person, they have complex and unfamiliar names that you can't avoid. We can only but mention them briefly here, with some degree of apology for their apparent complexity.

Some of the most notable phytochemicals being studied as 'active ingredients' in muscadine grapes include (but are not limited to):

Resveratrol	Myricetin	Catechin
Ellagic acid	Caffeic acid	Picaetannol
Quercetin	Epicatechin	Pectin fiber
Anthocyanidins	Gallic acid	Vitamin C
Kaempferol	Pterostilbene	OPC's
		(Oligomeric Procyanidins)

Many of these phytochemicals are well-known in the professional community and are being very actively studied. They have major **antioxidant** and **anti-inflammatory** effects and to appreciate the true power of muscadine grapes, we have to grapple with some of the details about these important natural ingredients.

Let's begin at the basics, to try to make some sense of what would otherwise be complex terminology. We'll use descriptive terms to make it easy.

Some people are familiar with the organic solvent, benzene. This has a 6-carbon ring structure and is the basis for most aromatic chemicals. Each of the carbon atoms has one hydrogen atom attached. If you substitute a hydrogen atom with a -OH hydroxyl group, you get a new molecule called *phenol*. All substances with a phenolic ring are then referred to as *phenolics*. When plant chemicals are analyzed by sophisticated methods, the total phenolic content identified and quantified becomes a useful measure of the presumed biological value of that plant (or alternatively, extracts or products derived from that plant). The analytical tests used for this purpose essentially measures the phenolic content, including every plant-based compound that contains a phenolic ring. Many of these are known to be protective of plants. That may have been their original purpose, but we have now learned that they greatly benefit human health as well.

Some phytochemicals have more than one phenol ring in their structure. They may be joined together in a variety of ways (usually by short chains of carbon atoms or other ring structures) to form what are called *polyphenolics*. This overall category would then contain some other important classes of biologically active molecules. Among them are the important bioflavonoids, including quercetin, catechins and epicatechin, anthocyanins, anthocyanidins, oligomeric proanthocyanidins (OPC's), stilbenes (including resveratrol) and ellagic acid. And that's just to name a few.

These **bioflavonoids** should be emphasized in particular. They derive from a backbone of chemicals called *chalcones* which contain two phenyl rings. These substances give plants much of their color and taste. In muscadines, they include cyanidins, catechin and epicatechin, quercetin and myricetin, among many others. These molecules have rather interesting and unique properties to excite many a chemist but suffice it to say here that they are all excellent antioxidants. Indeed bioflavonoids are most commonly known for their antioxidant capacity. However, more research has shown that the benefits they provide against cancer and heart disease are more likely the result of other mechanisms as well.

Bioflavonoids are quite varied and widely distributed. They have relatively low toxicity compared to other active plant compounds (like alkaloids) and humans do ingest significant quantities in fruits and vegetables. Some people refer to them as nature's *biological response modifiers'* since the evidence reveals their inherent ability to modify the body's reaction to allergens, viruses and carcinogens. They show anti-allergic, anti-inflammatory, anti-microbial and anti-cancer activity.

But the true situation is not yet clear. Recent results from the Linus Pauling Institute, published in the Journal *Free Radical Biology and Medicine,* suggest that bioflavonoids are poorly absorbed and quickly metabolized and excreted from the body, mainly via the biliary fecal route.[5] They themselves may not be the effective antioxidants but indirectly, from the increased uric acid levels that they produce. Further, they seem to induce so-called *Phase II enzymes* that secondarily help eliminate mutagens and carcinogens, which would account for their possible role in cancer prevention. They may even induce other mechanisms that help kill cancer cells and inhibit tumor invasion. Only small amounts of bioflavanoids are necessary for these dramatic results to be observed.

It is now generally accepted that many of the health benefits attributed to high intake of highly colored fruits and vegetables can reasonably be ascribed to this category of active phytochemicals.

Two important phytochemicals found in relative abundance in muscadines need to be highlighted. The first is **resveratrol.** This is the polyphenol that the media picked up on to help account for what is known as the "French Paradox'.

Essentially, the French Paradox refers to an observation, first made by the Irish physician Samuel Black back in 1819. He pointed out that the French consume a diet relatively rich in saturated fats, yet they suffer a relatively low incidence of coronary heart disease (CHD). Here's the more modern food consumption data from the F.A.O.:[6] The average French person consumed 108 gm per day of fat from animal sources in 2002, while the average American consumed 72 gm. The French eat four times as much butter, 60% more cheese and nearly three times as much pork. Although they consume only slightly more total fat, they do consume much more saturated fat (the bad fat!). However, data from the British Heart Foundation showed that in 1999, rates of death from CHD among males age 35-74 was 115 per 100,000 for people in the US, but only 83 per 100,000 in France.

Now, here's the kicker. The popular TV program *CBS 60 Minutes* aired a description of this paradox in the United States in 1991 and included the proposal that red wine, or alcohol, decreases the incidence of cardiac diseases. The theory was that one or more of the ingredients in red wine potentially helped the heart, and early clues pointed to *resveratrol.* That turned the spotlight on to red wine as a protection for the heart, around the world. Therefore, the sale and consumption of red wine noticably increased as a result.

Wine, particularly red wines, are indeed a source of resveratrol. But the associated health claim may have been a premature rush to judgment. Although research is continuing on resveratrol and there are significant health benefits to be derived as we will see later, the concentration in wine seems too low to account for the French Paradox. Other researchers now point to a different group of polyphenols called *oligomeric proanthrocyanidins (OPC's)*.[7] They believe that these active ingredients in red wine offer the greatest degree of protection to human blood-vessel cells. Further tests with 165 wines showed that these OPC's are found in greatest concentration in European red wines from certain areas, which does correlate with the longevity in these regions. Unlike resveratrol, the OPC's are present in red wine (and more so, in muscadines) in quantities that seem high enough to be significant. Still other hypotheses have been advocated to account for the French Paradox and the research continues.

Be all that as it may, resveratrol is a very important and bioactive phytochemical. **It is associated with a number of health benefits, such as anti-cancer, anti-viral, cardioprotective, anti-aging and anti-inflammatory effects, all of which have been demonstrated *in vitro* and reported in the scientific literature.** [8] Clinical trials *in vivo* are still in

24

progress.

Resveratrol is produced naturally by several plants when under attack by pathogens such as bacteria or fungi. In grapes, it is found primarily in the skin, but in muscadines it is also present in the seeds. In fact, the skins and seeds of muscadine grapes have about one hundred times the concentration of resveratrol as the pulp does. The amount found in grape skins varies considerably with the grape cultivar, it's geographic origin and exposure to fungal infection. In wine, the fermentation time is also important.

There is no comparison between muscadine wines and any other. Normal wine usually contains between 0.2 and 5.8 mg/L of resveratrol, depending on the grape variety. *White wines have much less since they are fermented after the skin has been removed.* Some wines produced from muscadine grapes contain up to 40 mg/L or more. Resveratrol nutritional supplements were originally sourced from ground, dried grape skins and seeds, but nowadays, a Japanese knotweed containing up to 187 mg/kg in the dried root is used as an economical, concentrated source.

The other noteworthy polyphenol to be highlighted here is called **ellagic acid.** This is another antioxidant found in numerous fruits and vegetables, including muscadine. In fact, this is one of the compounds in muscadines that distinguishes them from other grapes. *Ellagic acid and its many derivative forms, exist only in the muscadine and not to any significant amount in your typical supermarket grapes.*

Ellagic acid is found generally in tannin-bearing plants that produce a special category known as gallotannins. These become hydrolyzed by water to form ellagic acid and gallic acid. When ellagic acid combines with glucose in the plant, the water-soluble ellagitannins are formed. These are much more easily absorbed from the diet.

Research in cell cultures and lab animals has found that ellagic acid does slow the growth of some tumors caused by certain carcinogens. This is quite promising.[9] It has been found to cause apoptosis (cell death) in cancer cells in the lab and it can help the liver to break down or remove some cancer-causing substances from the blood. **It is an effective antioxidant**

and has been reported to reduce atherosclerosis and heart disease, birth defects, some liver problems and to promote wound healing.

Clearly, all that was said in the new *USDA Dietary Guidelines* about the value of consuming generous portions of fruits and vegetables as part of a balanced diet, will apply in spades to muscadines. Moreover, the additional value of important phytochemicals in muscadines, for all their antioxidant properties and much more, makes this a truly healthful addition to the best of diet regimens.

The phytochemicals in muscadines are indeed very powerful antioxidants, but how does one measure this and how can we make a comparison to anything else? The short answer is that there is now a standard assay to evaluate and compare antioxidants reliably and responsibly. It is called the *Oxygen Radical Absorbance Capacity* or ORAC test.

ORAC was originally developed by scientists at the National Institutes of Health. It essentially measures the oxidative degradation of a standard fluorescent molecule like flourescein, after being mixed with free radical generators (initiators), with or without the presence of the potential antioxidant. The initiators typically produce peroxy free radicals on heating, which damage the fluorescent molecules by an oxidation process, so that fluorescence decreases with time. Any antioxidant present should protect the fluorescent molecule from the oxidative degeneration. The corresponding degree of protection is quantified on a fluorometer. Automated ORAC equipment is now commercially available.

For purposes of standardization, a vitamin E analogue known as *Trolox*, a fairly good antioxidant itself, is commonly used as a standard of comparison. Different concentrations of Trolox are first used to make a standard curve, and test samples are then compared to this. Results from foods and other test samples are therefore commonly reported as 'trolox equivalents' or TE units. The method takes into account the fact that some samples have a lag phase to their antioxidant capacities. This is very applicable when measuring foods and food supplements that contain complex ingredients with various slow- and fast-acting antioxidants, as well as ingredients with combined effects that cannot be pre-calculated.

A wide variety of foods has been tested using this methodology and the highest ratings were found for berries, legumes and certain spices. Correlation between the high antioxidant (ORAC) capacity of fruits and vegetables, and the positive impact of diets high in fruits and vegetables, is believed to play an important role in the free-radical theories of many common diseases and the inevitable aging process.

Nevertheless, care should always be taken when comparing ORAC data. In particular here, attention must be given to the nature of the food (which berries?), its particular parts (whole berries, seeds, skins, juice, blends?), how processed (hot or cold? extracted in what medium?) and length of storage. Then the units may vary (per gram, per 100 gm, per serving size, per recommended dietary intake?). All these considerations make any *comparison* of ORAC values, implied antioxidant powers and associated nutraceutical benefits, a rather tenuous exercise.

ORAC values do measure the total antioxidant capacity derived from the total phenolic content of products such as those derived from muscadine. But it may also include the antioxidant effect of other antioxidants such as vitamin C. In principle, a product can indeed have a high ORAC value but little or no other phytochemicals, if it is simply spiked with vitamin C.

Having said all that, let's consider some real data for muscadine fractions and products. Typical ORAC values for whole muscadines range from about 23-66 units per gram of fresh fruit. This range overlaps the corresponding ranges for blueberries, blackberries, plums, oranges and grapefruit. That's for the whole berries in each case.

Muscadine berries consist of pulp, skins and seeds. The phenolic antioxidants and the geatest ORAC capacity are concentrated in the skins and seeds. The latter have proven to be excellent nutraceutical sources of antioxidants and polyphenolics. Here are the numbers: [10]

	ORAC (TE Units)
Fresh muscadine juice	5- 23 per lit
Fresh muscadine grapes	23- 66 per gm
Muscadine skins	422- 700 per gm
Muscadine seeds	667-1100 per gm

It is therefore obvious that the amount of total antioxidants in a gram of muscadine grape seeds is twice as much as in the grape skins, 10 times as much as in whole grapes, and at least 30 times as much as in the juice.

Take this a step further. Blueberries and blackberries are considered to be excellent choices in any daily fruit intake. They have ORAC values in the range of 52-139 TE units per gram and 2-82 units per gram respectively. Note that, in contrast, the muscadine seeds have more than 10 times as much antioxidant capacity as blueberries. There's no true comparison!

A comparison of the antioxidant capacities of some leading *functional beverages* on the market today is given in **Table 2**. These are all select blends derived principally from different grapes or berries, which are all claimed to be rich in nutraceuticals in general, and antioxidants, in particular. The results compare the ORAC scores, as well as the phenolic and anthocyanin content for these products (juice blends) derived from Muscadine grapes, Acai berries, Mangosteeen, and Goji berries. It also shows the results using two other standardized tests of the same antioxidant capacities, namely: the *Ferric Reducing Ability of Plasma* (FRAP) assay, and the *Trolox Equivalent Antioxidant Capacity* (TEAC) assay.

To help make the comparative picture clearer, the same ORAC data is illustrated more pictorially in the adjacent bar graph on page 30. All these *in vitro* test results were obtained by the world-class Brunswick Laboratories in Norton, MA. The results consistently show the exceptional antioxidant power of muscadine and why it is now justifiably perceived as **'the leader of the pack'**.

Here's the bottom line: **The best commercial juice blend or functional beverage derived from muscadine, provides about 2-4 times more antioxidant capacity per serving, than its popular competitors!**

Table. 2   A Comparison of Antioxidant Capacities

Blend ID	Brunswick Lab ID	ORAChydro* (µmoleTE/L)	Phenolics [1] (mg/L)	Anthocyanin [2]
Acai	08-0141	25,182	2,125.64	130.62
Mangosteen	08-0142	32,160	2,233.08	23.70
Goji	08-0143	14,874	1,516.84	ND
Muscadine	08-0144	63,647	3,532.10	238.87

* The ORAC analysis provides a measure of the scavenging capacity of antioxidants against the peroxyl radical, which is one of the most common reactive oxygen species (ROS) found in the body. ORAChydro reflects water-soluble antioxidant capacity. Trolox, a water-soluble Vitamin E ana-log, is used as the calibration standard and the ORAC result is expressed as micromole Trolox equivalent (TE) per liter.

[1]   The phenolic result is expressed as milligram gallic acid equivalent per liter.

[2]. The anthocyanin result is expressed as milligram cyanidine-3-glucoside equivalent per liter.

The acceptable precision of the ORAC assay is 15% relative standard deviation.

Blend ID Lab ID	Brunswick Lab ID	FRAP* (µmoleTE/L)	TEAC* (µmoleTE/L)
Acai	08-0141	11,474	27,738
Mangosteen	08-0142	12,114	34,181
Goji	08-0143	6,702	13,643
Muscadine	08-0144	25,189	59,743

Testing performed by H. Ji, J. Dion and J. Frietas, Brunswick Labs

A Graphical Comparison of Antioxidant Capacities
(µmol TE/L)

8. The Nutraceutical Value of Muscadines

We have been using the term 'nutraceutical' repeatedly in this monograph and unapologetically so. It is becoming quite a household word, thanks to the media and to the health food and food supplement industries. However, it's time to explore what this all means and why muscadines figure so prominently in this area.

It's less than a quarter century since this terminology was introduced. Dr. Stephen DeFelice coined the term for a presentation to a scientific meeting in Italy (1986):

*"**Nutraceutical** is the name I have given to a nutritional product - a single entity or combination which includes special diets - that reasonable clinical evidence has shown to have medical benefit that its manufacturer cannot claim to the public or the physician under present regulatory policy. Making a medical claim for a nutritional product makes that product a drug, according to the prevailing reasoning of the regulatory agency; claims made for drugs must be approved by the government."*

By its definition therefore, **any true nutraceutical will have some medical benefit** but no claims can be made for it. So there is an obvious paradox here. Once any food or food product is labeled a 'nutraceutical', the implication must be that its medical benefit exists, so claims are implied even though they cannot be explicitly stated. That hardly makes sense. We know there is benefit, but we cannot say there is benefit. It turns out, therefore, that what's good enough for science may not be good enough for sales, under the present regulations. However, education still has its place, and that's the objective here.

The FDA recognizes only 'dietary supplements' as defined by the Dietary Supplement Health and Education Act (DSHEA) passed in 1984. *A dietary supplement* is a product taken by mouth that contains a '*dietary ingredient*' included to supplement the diet. *Dietary ingredients* may then include: vitamins, minerals, herbs or other botanicals, amino acids and substances such as enzymes, organ tissues, glandulars and metabolites. Dietary Supplements can also be extracts or concentrates, and may be found in a variety of forms such as tablets, capsules, soft gels, gelcaps, liquids, or powders. They must be appropriately labeled, not as conventional foods or as sole items of a meal or diet. They do not need FDA approval to be marketed, but the manufacturer assumes responsibility for safety and adequate evidence to substantiate any representations or claims that are made about their products. **It is still illegal to promote and sell a dietary supplement as a treatment, prevention or cure for a specific disease or condition.**

Having said that, we again emphasize that our goal in this monograph is to educate the inquiring public about the inescapable value of muscadines as an excellent source of powerful phytochemicals that unquestionably affect the quality of health you can enjoy. Yet the science shows that they also impact the prevention and treatment of several medical conditions. But this should never be seen in isolation, since muscadines and the products derived from these healthful berries, make at best, a valuable contribution to any maximally healthy diet. Muscadines, or any other natural food or food supplement for that matter, should never be seen as a *substitute* for a normally adequate and balanced diet. They should never be presumed to be an *alternative* for any prescribed treatment or management option devised by a competent healthcare professional. But *they provide a remarkable complementary option* in the pursuit of optimum health. Of course, as a further disclaimer, we are quick to point out that none of these statements or conclusions have been evaluated by the US Food and Drug Administration.

Perhaps the best way to illustrate the real nutraceutical value of muscadines is simply to observe the intense level of research interest in the past decade. A mere ten years ago, there were but just a few scientific papers published on grape seed, grape seed extract and grape skin. Since then, there has been an almost exponential increase in the literature.

What's all the buzz about? Primarily it is about the powerful biological effects of the phenolic compounds found in such relative abundance in muscadine, especially in the seeds and skins. We can't say much about any specific commercial products *per se*, but we can inform the reader about the demonstrated value of these phenolic compounds in helping prevent and sometimes improve cases of heart disease and atherosclerosis, diabetes and metabolic syndrome, cancers, inflammatory disease, gastrointestinal diseases, neurological diseases and even the anti-aging phenomena being observed.

This subject has been well reviewed in an excellent monograph, Muscadine Medicine, by Diane K. Hartle, PhD, Phillip Greenspan PhD and James L. Hargrove PhD.[1]   For several years, these researchers have been conducting and publishing extensive research on muscadine grapes at the Nutraceutical Research Laboratory of the University of Georgia. Their proven results (among others) underline the scientific basis for the nutraceutical value of the muscadines and products derived from them.

More research is needed because there is a whole lot that we still do not know in this area. Present ideas are open to question and re-interpretation. But results to date are promising. Muscadines are precious natural fruits, with their best assets in the less palatable skins and seeds. When these are harnessed for convenience, by drying and pulverizing before packaging, one can derive maximum benefit from such concentrated sources. These particular concentrates deliver the real nutraceutical value of whole foods. The variety of phytochemicals remain in balance to deliver a synergistic bonus, unknown anywhere else but in nature.

Let's explore these health benefits some more.

9. The Health Benefits of Muscadine

Health is more than just the absence of disease. It is the presence of vital functions operating in the body, all in perfect unison and effective balance. Total health is the sum of all the individual healthy systems, each one doing its part with optimal efficiency. We refer to just four of these systems here.

9.1 Cardiovascular Health

The cardiovascular system refers to the heart and blood vessels (arteries and veins). The necessity of maintaining a healthy cardiovascular system cannot be overstated when you simply consider the statistics:

- Cardiovascular disease (CVD) is the leading cause of death and disability in the United States and Canada.

- CVD kills one person every 24 seconds in the US alone.

- Diseases of the heart alone cause 30% of all deaths, with other diseases of the cardiovascular system causing further substantial death and disability.

- Over 525,000 Americans die of coronary heart disease every year.

- Two out of every three cardio deaths occur without any diagnosis of CVD.

The underlying cause of most CVD is arterial disease (atherosclerosis) which is usually quite advanced by the time that heart problems are detected. In fact, the process of atherosclerosis evolves over decades and begins as early as childhood. A major study of young people aged 15-19 years demonstrated that intimal lesions had already appeared in the walls of all their aortas and more than half of their right coronary arteries. Those are delayed fuses, already ignited. Therefore, it is obvious that **in order to**

stem the tide of cardiovascular disease, primary prevention is needed.

When it comes to primary prevention, the identification of elevated risk factors is a reasonable starting point. Here is a Top 12 list in no specific order:

- Male gender   - Smoking   - Hypertension
- Poor diet   - Increasing age   - Diabetes
- Elevated homocysteine - Inordinate stress   - Positive family history
- High cholesterol   - Estrogen deficiency   -Sedentary lifestyle

Some of these factors cannot be modified (gender, age and family history) but there is great room for behavior modification and good medical management of relevant chronic conditions to alter the probable outcome in most individuals.

Research has clearly shown that dietary habits can decrease the risk of cardiovascular disease and increase normal life expectancy. Since the underlying cause of CVD is atherosclerosis, it is no surprise that **diet has major influences on the process by which plaque builds up in the vascular system.**

Let's just describe that process in general terms.

It begins at the surface of cells lining each blood vessel (endothelial cells). They interact with substances in the blood and with the smooth muscle cells and connective tissue cells that comprise the major part of the blood vessel wall. These endothelial cells partially regulate blood pressure, maintain proper blood clotting, and literally control the potential development of atherosclerotic plaque.

Think of the process in three steps, each of which is a malfunction of otherwise normal defensive physiology. The first step is one of **inflammation.** This is the body's normal response to injury and is designed to protect normal tissues by activating the immune system and summoning rescue workers, mainly *monocytes* initially (a type of white blood cell), to come to the site of damage or infection, to initiate normal repair and healing.

The endothelial lining may become chronically inflamed by a second step defined by high levels of **oxidation**. Several conditions make this high oxidative stress more likely and pronounced, including smoking, hypertension, diabetes, elevated LDL, elevated homocysteine levels and estrogen deficiency.

Oxidative stress damages the endothelial cells further. They begin to malfunction and some die (apoptosis). They summon more monocytes into the area which then hang around just inside the endothelial lining. The monocytes increase in size and become active scavengers called *macrophages*. These macrophages are then prone to trap some tiny particles in the blood, characterized by their low-density lipoprotein (LDL or bad cholesterol) content. More precisely, they trap the oxidized form or variant of the LDL particles. They ingest these particles (by phagocytosis) and thereby change their appearance to *'foam' cells*, as seen under the microscope.

The foam cells gradually increase in number and the cholesterol from the oxidized LDL continues to accumulate and build early *fatty streaks*. They also interfere with the adjacent smooth muscle cells causing some of them to change in form and function, into *'fibroblasts'*. These fibroblasts move into the plaque and do their thing, which is to synthesize fiber and collagen that provides scaffolding for the early plaque formation. When this activity surpasses the ability of the endothelial cells to maintain the integrity of the vessel lining, the underlying plaque erupts into the lumen where it is exposed directly to the blood. That activates the *platelets* (to arrest any potential blood loss) and a clot starts to form at the atherosclerotic site. This step we could call **precipitation.** Other chemicals released by the endothelial cells cause the vessel to constrict. Blood flow is now reduced and the stage is set for potential disaster.

So how could the phytochemicals in muscadines influence this descriptive **3-step process leading to atherosclerosis** and the dreaded consequences of cardiovascular disease?

In the first place, some polyphenolics in muscadines have been shown to have highly *anti-inflammatory properties*. That would potentially influence the first step. The details are beyond the scope of this monograph, but just to illustrate, we'll consider one mechanism by which this may happen.

As part of the inflammation process, monocytes and neutrophils (other white blood cells) are recruited, summoned to the activation site and kept there. To do this they are tagged by adhesion molecules on the cell surface, which are expressed only if certain genes are switched on. A known nuclear transcription factor (designated as *NF-kappa B*) powerfully regulates the expression of scores of genes associated with these *cell adhesion molecules* and *cytokines* involved in the inflammatory process. Now, here it comes - **phytochemicals in muscadines such as resveratrol, have been shown to inhibit the activation of NF-kappa B**. [11]

In the second step we outlined above, oxidative stress has a major impact on plaque formation. It reflects endothelial cell function, lipid deposition, vasoconstriction, smooth muscle cell activity and clot formation. Phenolic substances in muscadine are very potent antioxidants and therefore oppose each of those processes. Again, we cannot be exhaustive here, so we'll discuss just one mechanism that is known to involve the *antioxidant properties* of phytochemicals in muscadines.

We mentioned that oxidized LDL particles are more likely to become trapped in the atherosclerotic plaque. Naturally occurring Vitamin E and carotenoids in the LDL particles protect them from early oxidation but eventually they become susceptible. In particular, when one of their constituents (*apoliprotein B-100*) is oxidized, the particles can no longer bind to the special receptors necessary to remove cholesterol from the bloodstream. In laboratory tests, it has been found that catechins, quercetin, kaempferol, caffeic acid and p-coumaric acids - all phytochemicals found in muscadine - they all inhibit the oxidation of LDL. Purple grape juice has been shown to improve endothelial function while reducing the susceptibility of LDL to oxidation in patients. **Dietary consumption of flavonoids - powerful antioxidants - has been shown to be inversely related to morbidity and mortality from coronary heart disease.** [12]

In the third step which we labeled precipitation, the emphasis was on the formation of a clot in the area of atherosclerotic plaque. This could lead to vessel occlusion or embolism (clots breaking away and traveling in the blood stream).   Again, **phytochemicals in muscadine are known to influence this tendency for clots to form**. [13] Quercetin and resveratrol, in particular, both increase the production of enzymes that dissolve blood clots (namely, tissue plasminogen activator and tissue factor). They also block some of the triggers that cause blood to clot in the first place (such as the activation of thrombin and the aggregation of platelets).

It is clear just from these illustrative examples that muscadine grapes have a number of different phytochemicals that influence atherosclerosis, the underlying cause of cardiovascular disease. In a nutshell, they help to -

- Keep endothelial cells functioning properly;

- Reduce inflammation;

- Decrease the isolation of monocytes from the bloodstream;

- Keep LDL particles from becoming oxidized;

- Impede blood clotting and relax the vessel walls.

Reduction in atherosclerosis by any means would go a long way to easing the burden of cardiovascular disease. This would lead to fewer heart attacks and strokes, and let's not forget peripheral vascular disease which could also lead to much morbidity, if not death.

One further implication is worthy of mention, because it too refers to cardiovascular health. Endothelial cells produce an important messenger molecule called *nitric oxide*. This neglected molecule binds to the receptor sites of an enzyme called *guanylate cyclase* which results in increased levels of a metabolite called *cyclic guanosine monophosphate* (cGMP). This then leads to the relaxation of vascular smooth muscle, thereby widening the lumen, reducing the blood pressure and increasing the arterial blood flow.

This process just described affects the function of various vasculatures but few as important as the blood vessels that supply blood to the corpus cavernosum (the principal muscle of the penis). If the endothelical cells of those vessels cannot produce enough nitric oxide to cause them to expand, erectile dysfunction takes place. Phytochemicals - like the flavonoids, catechins, tannins and other **polyphenolics which are relatively abundant in muscadine grape skins and seeds - are believed to aid the endothelial cell function and its nitric oxide signaling pathway.** [14]

And that's not all, either. All over the media today, there are advertisements for drugs to improve erectile dysfunction. Who has not heard of Viagra,™ Levitron™ and Cialis™? These pharmaceuticals work by selectively inhibiting another enzyme called *cGMP specific phosphodiesterace* (PDES), which is responsible for the degradation of cGMP in the corpus cavernosum of the penis. That means more cGMP accumulates, and better erections ensue. Well, hold your breath - mixtures of grape skin anthocyanins (relatively abundant in muscadine) have also been shown to have similar excellent PDES inhibitors in the phenolic fraction.[15] Therefore, the phenolics in grapes can apparently both help to dilate the blood vessels of the penis and to protect the cells that line their lumens. What a potential bonus!

Cardiovascular disease in all its manifestations is a multifactoral condition. Flavonoids and other polyphenolics have been shown to be helpful in reducing oxidative stress associated with hypertension, diabetes, smoking, and elevated LDL. But each of these major risk factors for CVD requires a variety of interventions. **There is no substitute for healthy eating, exercise, avoidance of smoking and prudent management of any of these chronic medical conditions that increase CVD risk.**

Anyone concerned about their quality of life and health must address these issues. Diet must be a primary concern. All professionals agree on the importance of consuming low saturated fat, some calorie restriction, high fiber, essential fatty acids and not to be neglected, copious fruits and vegetables regularly. Perhaps, you now appreciate the value of all those dark purple fruits (rich in polyphenolics), and of muscadines in particular. Carefully processed muscadine products (especially of skins and seeds) would afford a more concentrated and convenient form of those essential bioactive ingredients. What a wise way to help protect your cardiovascular health!

9.2 **Chemoprevention and Cancer**

Just the mention of the 'C' word ('*Cancer*') speaks dread into the hearts and minds of most people. But not as much as it used to, thanks to advances in the three main modalities of treatment - chemotherapy, radiation therapy and surgery. We've come a long way from the early days when a diagnosis of cancer typically meant an almost inevitable, early fatal prognosis. In fact, for a few types of cancer, the five and ten year survival rates can surpass 90% particularly with early diagnosis and good medical management.

However, there is no getting around it. Most types of cancer will make a profound impact in any person's life. Their prognosis will depend not only on the type of cancer, but also on the stage or extent of the disease.

The impressions on the public's mind is so influenced (if not controlled) by the media. Some high profile personalities in the media who have rebounded from cancer, resumed active life and even taken on arduous athletic challenges, offer increasing hope to the general population. But cancer can strike anyone at any age. **In the US and other developed countries, cancer is presently responsible for about 25 percent (1 in 4) of all deaths.** On a yearly basis, 0.5 percent (1 in 200) of the population is diagnosed with cancer. In men, the three most common by occurrence are: prostate (33%), lung (13%) and colorectal (10%); compared to those in women: breast (32%), lung (12%) and colorectal (11%). In terms of mortality, lung cancer tops the list in either case.

The actual causes of cancer are many and varied and not always identifiable. We do know that some are clearly influenced by hereditary factors, since an immediate family history of cancer usually increases the relative chances for other members of that family. But clearly, exposure to environmental factors - including diet, tobacco smoke and chemicals in the environment, some infectious agents and radiation - also plays a major role. The common thread in all known cancers is the acquisition of abnormalities in the genetic material of the cancer cell and its progeny (those formed as it multiplies). Different agents and events cause or facilitate genetic changes in cells that are then destined to become cancerous. This group of cells then display the characteristic traits of *uncontrolled growth* (they grow and divide beyond normal limits), *invasion* (they intrude and destroy adjacent tissues) and, left to themselves, they sometimes show *metastasis* (they spread to other locations in the body via the lymph or blood).

Since cancer is cellular in origin, the abnormalities in the genetic material that causes normal cells to become cancerous is of fundamental importance. We now understand that genes control cell growth and replication, and two classes of genes are considered critical. First, cancer-promoting *oncogenes* can be *activated* to give prospective cancer cells new and unusual properties: hyperactive growth and division, protection against their programmed cell death, and loss of respect for normal tissue boundaries. On the other hand, *tumor suppression genes* can be *inactivated* to cause cancer cells to lose their normal capacity for: accurate DNA replication, control over the cell cycle, orientation and adhesion within tissues, and interaction with protective cells of the immune system.

Much research is going on around the world on all aspects of cancer, especially its probable causes and potential cures.

The National Cancer Institute (NCI) champions all these research endeavors but still makes the possible *prevention of cancer* its highest priority. And when it comes to that - no question about it - **dietary considerations have a major impact on cancer risk.** However, diet is not everything, so we must mention other potentially modifiable risk factors like: tobacco smoking, excessive alcohol use, limited physical exercise, HPV infection (irresponsible or unsafe sex), urban air pollution, infections (hepatitis B and C), use of exogenous hormones, chemical exposure in the workplace, and obesity.

This booklet is about diet and dietary supplements, in particular, so we must emphasize that **diets low in fruits and vegetables represent a significant risk factor.** And there are many other dietary factors to consider - for example, *reduced meat consumption* (especially grilled meat) is associated with decreased risk of colon cancer, among others. Many studies have suggested a role for *vitamins* in cancer prevention. *High fiber* diets have also been demonstrated to protect against gastro-intestinal cancers. And the list goes on.

As far as fruit and vegetables are concerned, and their important role in cancer prevention, there is no real debate. We now know that phytochemicals found in these foods are highly protective against different types of premature oxidation that contribute to the beginnings of cancer. This is an example of what is termed '*chemoprevention*' or chemoprophylaxis. This new concept may be defined in layman's terms as *the use of any food, drug or dietary supplement to help prevent the incidence, increase, or spread of any disease.* This is true primary prevention and in this area of cancer, the polyphenolics such as are found in the muscadines lead the way. On the one hand, the NCI warns that long term, poor dietary habits support or cause a large proportion of various types of cancer. On the other hand, they promote a high intake of fruits and vegetables, with a wide spectrum of phytochemicals, to help to prevent various cancer types.

There's just too much information on the role of antioxidants in general, and natural polyphenolics in particular, with respect to cancer chemoprevention, to do this subject any justice here. We will therefore zero-in on three specific phytochemicals - all found in muscadines, especially - that have been researched the most and have been demonstrated to have anti-cancer properties. We'll consider ellagic acid, resveratrol and quercitin, in that order.

Ellagic acid, you recall, is one of the powerful polyphenolic antioxidants in the muscadines. It is also present in other foods like raspberries, blueberries, cranberries, pecans, walnuts and pomegranates. Researchers at Ohio State University have led this area of research.[16] They demonstrated unequivocally - first in the laboratory with *in vitro* tests, then *in vivo* with animal models and finally in *clinical trials* with humans - that ellagic acid is an effective agent for chemoprevention of cancer. They used synthetic ellagic acid, then its naturally occurring forms and finally, fruit extracts containing ellagic acid and other phenolics. They looked at animal models for esophageal cancer, colon cancer and lung cancer.

The conclusions from this type of on-going research suggest that ellagic acid is active at the different stages of cancer. Different research groups were able to demonstrate, for example, that ellagic acid prevented the initiation of many different cancer types in rodents exposed to a wide variety of well-known carcinogens.[17] More specifically, it was found that ellagic acid, as a powerful antioxidant, induces the gene expression of the *QR enzyme* which is active in the detoxification of many carcinogens.

In some cases where test systems of cancer cells were exposed to ellagic acid, the rate of proliferation was substantially reduced. Those results were consistent for cancers of the colon, breast and prostate. Ellagic acid impairs the formation of new blood vessels that necessarily must grow in to feed some solid tumors. It arrests the cell cycle, inhibits overall cell growth and induces cell death (apoptosis) in cervical cancer cells.

Since ellagic acid is poorly absorbed through the intestine, it is important to note that *in vivo*, its effect would most likely be most pronounced inside the gastrointestinal tract where it could come into direct contact with the epithelial surface. It would therefore be expected to suppress cancers of the mouth, esophagus, stomach, small intestine and colon. Somewhat surprisingly, it has been shown that the epithelial cells lining the gut actually concentrate ellagic acid.

In summary, although much more research needs to be done, it does appear that **ellagic acid - a known significant phytochemical in muscadines - does inhibit the activation of some known redox-sensitive transcription factors that regulate gene expression.** [18] Some of these genes help to enhance the progression of the cell cycle which is needed for cancer cells to proliferate.

A second important polyphenol in muscadine that has received much attention as a chemoprotective agent is **resveratrol**. Its activity in some ways is very similar to ellagic acid. It similarly inhibits all three major phases of carcinogenesis: initiation, promotion and progression. Even some of the mechanisms of action are similar. For example, resveratrol inhibits genes that express a system of enzyme proteins known as *cytochrome P450* that can convert different chemicals and metabolites into carcinogens.[19] It also induces some *Phase II enzymes* that help convert possible mutagens into harmless chemicals. And that's only the beginning.

Resveratrol helps to regulate the cell cycle. In particular, when normal cells undergo DNA mutations that convert them into possible cancer cells, resveratrol has the ability to induce mechanisms that stop these cells from growing and proliferating.[20] In fact, it can cause these cells to die a targeted or programmed death - a phenomenon that scientists call *apoptosis*.

There is yet more. Resveratrol has been shown to down regulate the gene expression of enzymes that cancer cells use to downgrade their environment as they create space for growth and proliferation.[21] Like other polyphenolics in muscadines, resveratrol is also an *angiogenisis inhibitor.*[22] That means that it blocks signals between tumor cells and blood vessel cells, so that new blood vessels do not grow well into the tumor to feed its growth.

Like ellagic acid, resveratrol you recall, also tends to have poor bioavailability. It is therefore not surprising that the best **chemoprevention is likely to be seen from topical application (skin tumors) and cancers of the gastro-intestinal tract.** Results bear this out. Resveratrol has been shown to inhibit skin damage and decrease skin cancer in mice, when applied both before and after ultraviolet exposure. It also prevented or reduced esophageal, intestinal and colon cancer, again in mice.[23]

A third bioflavanoid in the muscadine repertoire should not be left out. That is **quercetin,** another potent antioxidant and anti-inflammatory agent. In some studies, this active ingredient is found to be the most potent, compared to other bioflavanoids, and some researchers contend that many nutraceutical plants owe much of their activity to their high quercetin content. This is obviously only partly true of muscadines, considering the competition from many other polyphenolics. But muscadines could represent a good source of quercetin intake.

However, quercetin has earned its reputation as a nutraceutical and among other things, it shows anti-tumor properties. It protects against DNA mutations and colon cancer. One study in the *British Journal of Cancer* shows that, when treated with a combination of quercetin and ultrasound for one minute, skin and prostate cancer cells showed a 90% mortality within 48 hours, with no visible mortality of normal cells.[24]

All that is only the tip of an iceberg. Muscadines contain not just ellagic acid, resveratrol and quercitin. There are many other bioflavanoids (or more generally, polyphenolics) in these purple grapes that are known to have anti-cancer properties.

We have not even mentioned the role of catechins, anthocyanins and proanthocyanidins in chemoprevention of cancer. But the idea is that once you realize the benefit of just one or two of the potent antioxidants in muscadines, then it makes sense to add the value of concentrated muscadine products to your dietary supplement regime. You will be rewarded with *all* the possible benefits of *all* the nutraceuticals present in the natural berries. That's what nature does, yielding much more benefit than you expect at any time.

9.3 Controlling Sugar

There is no doubt about it, diabetes is clearly in the **Top 10** and perhaps the **Top 5**, of the most significant diseases in the developed world. It is gaining in significance, not only in North America and Europe but also now in Asia and Africa, where it is expected that by about 2030, the majority of cases will then be found.

Here in North America, the prevalence of diabetes is now being called an epidemic by the CDC in Atlanta. Just consider the following statistics:

- There were 20.8 million people with diabetes in the US in 2005.

- Add an estimated 6.2 million undiagnosed with the disease, and another 41 million considered prediabetic.

- It is estimated that 1 in 3 Americans born after 2000 will develop diabetes in their lifetime.

- The number of pregnant American women with diabetes has doubled in the past 6 years.

- For Americans age 60 and older, 1 in 6 have diabetes.

- Diabetes costs exceed $130 billion each year in the US.

Those are staggering statistics that should make controlling blood sugar a high priority in health promotion and medical care. **Any intervention that can help the individual at risk for diabetes and its possible complications is worthy of consideration.**

Diabetes itself (specifically, the most common *diabetes mellitus*) is a syndrome characterized by disordered metabolism and abnormally high blood sugar. This results from insufficient levels of the insulin hormone, with or without additional resistance to insulin's effects in many body cells. Classically, Type I patients don't make enough insulin because of a deficiency in *production* in the cells of the pancreas, whereas Type II patients have problems *responding* to the insulin that is made - a type of insulin resistance.

Sometimes diabetics are only discovered when they have acute illness that takes them to the emergency room, or when they develop complications from end organ damage. These complications may involve coronary artery disease (angina); eye problems (blurring of vision due to cataracts or retinal changes); kidney problems (urinary changes, including sugar in the urine, to acute renal failure); peripheral vascular insufficiency (pain in the legs); nerve problems (tingling or loss of sensation in the feet); or poor wound healing (sores and ulcers).

But that need not be so. Common symptoms of poor sugar control are: increased frequency and volume of urination (*polyuria*), increased thirst and fluid intake (*polydypsia*), increased appetite (*polyphagia*), and unexplained *weight loss*. Any of these should be reported to the doctor who can confirm the diagnosis of diabetes with simple blood and urine tests.

Diabetes is not uncommonly seen in a cluster of metabolic characteristics now referred to as **metabolic syndrome.** This syndrome groups together patients who are diabetic or prediabetic, but also tend to have a poor lipid profile (high cholesterol, especially with low HDL, and high triglycerides), as well as abnormal obesity and often, hypertension. This cluster of symptoms is in epidemic proportions in affluent societies like America, where it is estimated that up to 25% of the population is now afflicted.

Both diabetes (mainly Type II) and metabolic syndrome are known to be influenced by lifestyle and environmental factors. Diet and exercise, in particular, are both crucial factors. In both cases, we know that decreasing calorie intake (especially from simple, refined sugars) and increasing physical exercise, go a long way to causing intentional weight loss, improving blood sugar control and generally reducing symptoms of disease. When these lifestyle interventions prove inadequate for the relief of chronic conditions, the next management approach of most doctors involves the use of drugs to control blood sugar, cholesterol and triglycerides, and blood pressure where necessary.

That's all basic background to what really concerns us here. Muscadines we have already seen, are loaded with important phytochemicals that have beneficial effects in many areas of human health. It's no surprise that some of these active natural ingredients also impact both the incidence of abnormal glucose control in the blood and its consequences. Taken together, the research shows that **phytochemicals in muscadine can help** in these areas by any or all of the following:

- Decreasing blood glucose levels

- Enhancing the action of insulin hormone

- Reducing resistance to insulin

- Protecting large blood vessels

- Preserving the integrity of small capillaries

- Reducing oxidative stress

- Reducing inflammation

- Opposing the oxidation of LDL cholesterol

- Lowering blood pressure by relaxing blood vessels

That's quite an impressive list, and there are hundreds of published reports to substantiate the beneficial effects of the muscadine phytochemicals on blood glucose control and on some other effects of diabetes. Flavonoids and other polyphenols in grape seeds and skins slow sugar absorption from the intestines, increase the activity of insulin and generally tend to reduce blood sugar.[25]

It is rather interesting to observe that something like muscadine, which has a rather sweet-tasting juice, could in fact be beneficial to diabetics. But it really is. The sweet taste is derived from the natural combination of fructose (the fruit sugar), glucose and some sucrose, but in the right combination with everything else to cause it to have a low glycemic index. It does not spike glucose levels by rapid absorption as in the consumption of simple refined sugar. There is no evidence that pure muscadine juice is unsafe, or even undesirable for diabetic patients.

Furthermore, the most important phytochemicals that help regulate blood glucose levels are more concentrated in the seeds and skins, where there is even less sugar, and there is much more benefit to be derived.

Consider the potential complications of diabetes. It is believed that most of these are derived from the increased reaction of glucose and fructose with the amine ligands of some amino acids that make up the proteins in different tissue structures. That produces *advanced glycosylation end products* (AGE). These are formed inside the walls of blood vessels when and where sugar levels are elevated. This can facilitate the development of plaque formation and over time, lead to end-organ damage. AGE proteins are implicated in the long-term potential damage of the eyes, kidneys, and nerves in diabetics.

Again, the good news is that the type of phytochemicals found in the muscadines, especially in the seeds and skins, appear to block the same glycation of proteins by sugars in the blood.[26]

In a different mechanism, glucose can be converted to fructose via a sorbitol intermediate. This so-called, *polyol pathway* produces reactive oxygen species leading to increased oxidative stress, increased AGE products as before, and more osmotic stress. There is then a tendency to elevate blood pressure. All of this can lead to tissue injury. The enzyme that converts glucose to sorbitol in the first and rate-limiting step of this polyol pathway is called *aldose reductase* and guess what? Muscadines again contain several phytochemicals that effectively inhibit this key enzyme, aldose reductase.[27] Ellagic acid, quercetin, myricetin, kaempferol and others can get the job done. Some of them even appear to go a step further and inhibit the action of nuclear transcription factors involved in the gene expression of that same enzyme.[28]

What's the bottom line? Muscadine is by no means a cure for diabetes. It simply is not. But anyone who is concerned about blood sugar control - whether they are diabetic, prediabetic, obese or having the metabolic syndrome - should consider the value of this natural intervention. **A daily intake of the important phytochemicals, preferably as natural concentrates from muscadine grapes, can only help to improve blood sugar control and may even help to reduce the possibility of end-organ complications, long term.** This is only complementary, however, to other useful lifestyle interventions of proper diet, exercise, stress management, and the use of oral hypoglycemics or insulin, where necessary to achieve adequate blood sugar control. It is always wise to consider nutraceuticals as *complementary* to all other good lifestyle choices, to any other professional care, and certainly not as first-line alternative where medical management is obviously indicated.

Helping to control blood sugar is just one more health benefit to be derived from this precious muscadine source.

9.4 Controlling Inflammation

By now you have come to appreciate the exceptional value of the powerful anti-oxidant properties of many phytochemicals found in muscadines. This is a major factor that contributes to the remarkable health benefits of this all-American grape. We've seen the protection that it affords against cardiovascular disease, cancer and hyperglycemia. That is by no means the whole story of this emerging nutraceutical source. In addition to the antioxidant properties of these natural ingredients, we turn next to emphasize their anti-inflammatory role. We have only alluded to it in passing until now. But this potential function in the body is critical.

To put it simply, *inflammation is the body's normal response to injury.*

More pointedly, it is a complex biological response of vascular tissues to harmful injury or insult, such as pathogens (disease causing organisms), damaged cells, or irritants. Whenever such exposure takes place, from whatever cause or source, the body responds in kind by seeking to isolate and remove the harmful stimulus, and then begin the healing or recovery process. Just imagine what would happen if the body did not have this major line of self defense. Then bleeding would not stop, wounds would not heal, infection would spread and ... the individual would eventually die. Inflammation can therefore be a life-saving response, and in many cases, it really is.

But on the other extreme, what if the body got its cues wrong and failed to identify injury and insult appropriately? What if the system responded to normal cells and tissues as if they were 'the enemy' and started to mount inflammatory response where none was really called for? Then a host of allergic and *autoimmune* conditions would ensue. Then you could suffer from a host of diseases, from simple hay fever to lupus, or from athero-sclerosis to rheumatoid arthritis, just to name a few. There are numerous auto-immune conditions where the body seems to fight against itself. Therefore, inflammation is a balancing act between adequate *defense* against external injury or cellular rebellion through mutation, on one hand, and the inordinate *offense* against otherwise normal tissue, on the other. For this reason, **inflammation is usually tightly regulated by the body**.

In the broadest terms, inflammation is classified as either acute or chronic and the difference is quite significant. *Acute inflammation* refers to the ini-tial response of the body to any harmful stimulus whereby there is increased blood flow to the active site. Plasma and leukocytes (white blood cells) move from the blood into surrounding tissues. Then follows an interesting cascade of biochemical events that involve the local vascu-lar system, the immune system and various tissue cells. The immediate result leads to *redness* and *heat* (from increased blood flow), *swelling* (from extravasation of the plasma into surrounding tissue), *pain* (from tis-sue distension and nerve end compression), and soon *declining function*. The white blood cells crowd the tissue spaces, help to wall off the insult and begin the mop-up operations. When the acute inflammation subsides, the damaged tissue is essentially repaired. Of course, depending on the severity of the challenge and the particular tissues involved, the repair may be partial or complete, with or without residual scarring.

If the inflammatory process is prolonged, usually by persistent or recurrent insult, then *chronic inflammation* sets in. There is a progressive shift in the type of cells utilized at the active site and the process involves *simultaneous destruction and healing* of the surrounding tissues. The characteristic 'acute' signs are not necessarily present but there is constant recruitment of mononuclear immune cells to do the on-going work of defense. It becomes a protracted operation.

The inflammation process has been intensively studied for many years and even today, it remains at the forefront of most investigations of pathophysiology (the origins of disease processes). We cannot begin to elucidate the complex 'control and communication' operations that define inflammation. Suffice it to say that there are very important cascade systems such as:

- The *complement* system for assisting and removing pathogens.

- The *kinin* system for sustaining blood flow and supplies.

- The *coagulation* system for covering the site of injury.

- The *fibronolysis* system for limiting the clotting system.

All these cascade systems and the operations of the front-line cells at the inflammation site are controlled by effective mediators, derived *either* from the plasma (e.g. bradykinin, complement proteins, membrane attack complex, plasmin, thrombin) *or* from participating cells (e.g. enzymes, histamine, interferons, prostaglandins, tissue necrosis factor, interleukins, nitric oxide, leukotriene). These cellular factors are called *cytokines*, which get into the circulation and cause pain and havoc in different parts of the body. When inflammation takes place, there is also an increase in the blood levels of what are called *acute-phase proteins*. These include, in particular, C-reactive protein, amyloid A, homocysteine and fibrinogen, which are sometimes markers (blood tests) for levels of inflammation in the body. There is also quite often an increased level of white blood cells, although in some cases there could be a marked decrease.

Now to the issue at hand with muscadine, as a source of **anti-inflammatory power**. As we have said, the antioxidant effect of phytochemicals found in muscadine can help to reduce 'oxidative stress' which is itself a major cause of local and systemic inflammation. That is one way in which muscadine can reduce inflammation. But there is good evidence that phytochemicals in muscadines are not just anti-oxidants but they are directly anti-inflammatory.

For example, when human monocytes were grown in the laboratory and then treated with a drug (called LPS) to stimulate inflammation, those cells released a powerful chemical, called prostaglandin (PGF2), a major mediator of inflammation. However, when muscadine extract was present, the inflammatory response was inhibited and more importantly, in a dose-dependent fashion.[29] This all happened at levels of dilution of the extract where there were even less phytochemicals present than what is found in whole muscadines, muscadine juice, wine or food supplements.

In other experiments, muscadine skins have been shown to inhibit the release of cytokines by activated human mononuclear cells, and the release of superoxide free radicals by activated neutrophils.[30] The results were again concentration-dependent. They were not unlike the effect of aspirin, a different kind of celebrated anti-inflammatory agent.

Those were all *in vitro* (test tube) experiments. Results with small mammals (rats) also confirm the anti-inflammatory power of muscadine *in vivo*. Male rats were fed whole muscadine skin powder as part of their diet for a couple weeks and then infected with carrageenan (a standard for this purpose) to cause inflammatory swelling (edema) in a hind paw. Three hours later they had 50% less paw edema than the controls.[31] Again, this demonstrated the anti-inflammatory power of muscadine at work.

The drugs that are normally used to counter inflammation are basically steroids or non-steroidals (NSAIDS). The corticosteroids reduce inflammation or swelling by binding to cortisol receptors. By a different mechanism, the NSAIDS (like aspirin, ibuprofen and naproxen) alleviate pain by counteracting an enxyme called *cyclooxygenase* (or COX II). This enzyme converts arachadonic acid from tissue breakdown into prostaglandins which are strong mediators of inflammation. Then there is the other enzyme called *lipoxygenase* (or LOX) which converts the same arachadonic acid into leukotrienes which are key to some inflammatory diseases (like asthma).

Here's more good news about muscadines. **A number of phytochemicals in muscadines have been shown to inhibit either COX II or LOX.**[32] These include some we've mentioned before like kaempferol, myricetin, OPC's, epicatechin, quercetin and resveratrol.

One more anti-inflammatory mechanism for muscadine phytochemicals should be enough. We mentioned that in the inflammatory process, white cells adhere to the blood vessel walls at the active site and make their way across into the tissue, along with the extravasating plasma. This part of the overall process is more complex that it might appear. When the endothelial cells are activated, they express binding proteins called *selectins*. The white blood cells have corresponding receptors called *integrins* on their surfaces and needless to say, they both get it together. Finally, the white cells can pass through, between the endothelial cells that line the blood vessel wall. That's called *trans migration.*

The key here is that those cell adhesion molecules which facilitate the above mechanism, are expressed by genes activated by the same NF-kappa B factor that was mentioned earlier. **Inhibition of this NF-kappa B, which includes phytochemicals from the muscadines, can limit the transmigration of the white cells which is a critical step in the inflammation process.** [33] The same transmigration process is also important in many inflammatory diseases, and in cancer metastasis as well.

Muscadines represent an excellent source of nutraceuticals. They have effective anti-inflammatory action, but they are not drugs. They do help to suppress activation of the vascular endothelial cells. They do reduce gene expression for cell adhesion molecules. They do decrease cytokine signaling molecules. They do reduce oxidative stress. All these effects and more, qualify them for a significant role in reducing unwanted inflammation especially chronic inflammation. But in cases where this therapeutic effect proves inadequate, then and perhaps only then, one should resort to more powerful anti-inflammatories, knowing that the increased side effects of those drugs would always be the price one has to pay.

10.   CONCLUSION

Healthy Aging

People are living longer. Normal life expectancy has reached 77-80 years of age in North America (up from only 47 in 1900). In addition, the baby boomer generation (born between 1946-64) represents a significant cohort of individuals now in midlife and beyond, that will soon make the category of 'seniors' a more prevalent and significant group in society.

But life expectancy is only one measure of prognosis. It focuses on the length of life - in other words, the *quantity of life*. The other measure is just as important, where you consider the *quality of life*. What kind of lifestyle could you enjoy in your later years? Would there be chronic illness with significant morbidity, or could you remain active and healthy even long into retirement?

Both the quantity and quality of life can be drastically affected by a host of factors which include gender, genetics, access to quality healthcare, hygiene, diet and nutrition, exercise, lifestyle and crime rates. The net effect is a present trend toward both increasing the quantity and improving the quality of life in North America.

> You can add up to ten years to your normal lifespan by eating right, engaging in useful exercise and avoiding unnecessary risks.

But recent increases in the rates of lifestyle diseases - such as obesity (recall, now an epidemic in the US), diabetes, hypertension and heart disease - may drastically slow down or even reverse this trend. In the other direction, we also know that you can add up to ten additional years to your normal lifespan by just eating right, engaging in useful physical exercise and avoiding unnecessary risks.

It's probably fair to suggest that most people today would emphasize the quality of life above its quantity. People would be prepared to age if they must, but to do so only with grace, good cognition and some measure of healthy enjoyment. Therefore, when all is said and done, the risks of chronic disease becomes the major focus.

There's no doubt about it. The quality of life you will lead as you get older will reflect very much on the kind of lifestyle you adopt today. You can choose to place strong emphasis on exercise, adequate sleep and relaxation skills, managing stress, emotional intimacy and most of all, proper diet and dietary supplementation. You need not become fanatical about weight training, grueling sports or running marathons. But you must pay attention to all the dietary choices you make. If you wish to look good, feel good, and live as long as you possibly can, then nutrition and supplementation must be a high priority.

Everyone agrees that there is great health benefit to be derived from a diet rich in fresh fruits and vegetables. Several daily servings in this category feature prominently in the new USDA Dietary Guidelines, and rightly so. But the benefits to be derived, primarily

The potential value of muscadines in health and disease can hardly be overemphasized.

from the rich phytochemical content of these foods, can be maximized by including copious portions of muscadine grapes or other more concentrated muscadine products, and with good justification, as we will now see.

We have already seen the value of muscadine phytochemicals in helping to protect the heart and blood vessels. We also observed a role for muscadines in helping to prevent some cancers. Then we looked at the value of these same polyphenolics as active muscadine ingredients that help to regulate blood sugar, and help to reduce chronic inflammation and its associated diseases. **These same nutraceuticals, acting primarily as antioxidants and anti-inflammatory agents, can go a long way in defending the human body against the morbidity of all these prevalent chronic diseases that greatly reduce the quality of life, especially in later years**. In fact, as a further observation, these conditions just mentioned account for the majority of all deaths in North America. So the potential value of muscadines in health and disease can hardly be overemphasized. And yet there is more.

Some researchers have been focused on the so-called 'aging process' in hope of gaining more understanding, and perhaps even some practical strategies for possible life extension. Studies with laboratory animals clearly demonstrated that reducing caloric intake by 30-40% (but maintaining other essential nutrients), reduced heart disease and cancer, while increasing overall life span.[34] Such dietary restrictions seem to defend the brain against the normal effects of oxidative stress, which itself tends to increase with age. But other antioxidants (like vitamins C and E, and selenium) are not so effective. There is clearly also an effect on the brain's stress-related genes. Other factors like local inflammation, calcium release from dead brain cells and tiny hemorrhages are also involved in the aging process in the brain.

But the best hope of dietary intervention to increase the quality of life or normal lifespan, comes again from the effects of nutraceuticals found in some berries (especially muscadines) and leafy green vegetables like spinach. When laboratory animals are fed a diet with 1-2% dried berries or spinach, for example, they clearly have significantly increased normal lifespan.[35] The effect is believed to be due to the antioxidant effects of polyphenolics, especially some of the anthocyanins that have been shown to actually enter the brain. You will recall that these same anthocyanins give the rich color to muscadine grapes, especially the dark purple variety. Blueberries have them too, as the media has popularized, but muscadines get the first prize.

There may also be indirect effects of the muscadine phytochemicals. Recall the master intracellular antioxidant called glutathione that we discussed earlier. Well, it appears that some plant polyphenolics (e.g. quercetin) can activate the gene that encodes for the enzyme responsible for making glutathione inside the cell.[36] Again, that's often the way with nature. Cooperate and you will get, surprisingly, more than you bargain for.

Speaking of that, let's just mention one more bonus, in conclusion. Everyone is familiar with the crucial role of DNA in cellular reproduction. Damaged DNA (by whatever method) can give rise to mutations which lead to disease, especially cancers. There is a family of proteins known as *sirtuins*, which are crucial in the usual repair mechanisms that avoid accumulation of incidental DNA mutations. These proteins can be blocked by a protein they produce (called NAD). However, some of the polyphenolics found in muscadine grapes (eg. resveratrol or quercetin) can disinhibit the sirtuins so that they remain active, facilitate DNA repair, and thereby help cells to live longer.[37]

Enough. It is clear that **muscadines will go a long way to help protect cells from premature oxidation and inflammation.** From all the evidence to date, the powerful nutraceutical value of these grapes makes them a superlative choice in the pursuit of not just the quality of health you enjoy, but perhaps also the quantity of your normal lifespan, all other things being equal.

Therefore, give a salute to Muscadines, the amazing berries now proven to be **America's Number One Source of Nutraceuticals.** They are packed with powerful phytochemicals which have amazing antioxidant and anti-inflammatory effects and much, much more ... to benefit your health ... today and tomorrow.

Salute!!

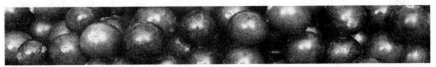

Selected References

1. Hartle DH, Greenspan P, Hargrove JL, Muscadine Medicine, Blue Heron Nutraceuticals, LLC, 2005, 128 pgs., 482 refs.
2. For general reading, see Muscadine Grapes, Edited by Basionny FM, Himelrick DG, ASHS Press, Alexandria VA, 2001, 378 pgs.
3. United States Department of Agriculture - Dietary Guidelines, 2005. See http://www.pyramid.gov/guidelines/index.html.
4. Ector BJ, Welch AS, Harkness E, Hegwood CP: "Nutritional components of red muscadine grapes: Levels of protein, carbohydrate, fat, dietary fiber, pectin and selected minerals and vita-mins." In: *Southern Assoc Agric Scientists, Food Sci Human Nutr Sec*: 1993; 1993: 32.
5. Lotito SB and Frei B, "Consumption of flavonoid-rich foods and increased plasma antioxidant capacity in humans: cause, consequence or epiphenomenon?" *Free Radic. Biol. Med.*, 2006, 41 (12): 1727-46.
6. See http://en.wikipedia.org/wiki/french_paradox.
7. "Procyanidins may be the factor behind red wine's cardioprotective effect." *Nature*, 2006, 444:566.
8. a) Delmas D, Lancon A, Colin D, Jannin B, Latruffe N, "Resveratrol as a chemopreventive agent: a promising molecule for fighting cancer," *Current Drug Targets 2006, (4):423-42.*
   b) Palamara AT, Nencioini L, Aquilano K, et al, "Inhibition of influenza and virus replication by resveratrol." *Journal of Infectious Diseases,* 2005, 191 (10): 1719-29.
   c) Wu JM, Wang ZR, Hsich TC, Bruder JL, Zou JG, Huang YA: Mechnism of cardioprotection by resveratrol, a phenolic antioxidant present in red wine (Review). *Int J Mol Med* 2001, 8(1): 3-17.
   d) Baur JA et al. "Resveratrol improves health and survival of mice on a high calorie diet." *Nature*, 2006, 444: 337-342
   e) de la Lastra CA, Villegas I: "Resveratrol as an anti-inflammatory and anti-aging agent: mech-anisms and clinical implications." *Mol Nutr Food Res* 2005, 49 (5): 405-430.
9. Mandals, Stoner GD. "Inhibition of N-nitrosobenzylmethylamine - induced esophageal tumori-genesis in rats by ellagic acid." *Carcinogenesis*, 1990, 11:55-61.
10. Morris JR, Brady PL: "The Muscadine Experience. Adding Value to Enhance Profits".*Arkansas Agricultural Experiment Station Research Reports* 2004, 974: 1-80.
11. Kundu JK, Surh YJ: "Molecular basis of chemoprevention by resveratrol: NF-kappaB and AP-1 as potential targets." *Mutat Res* 2004, 555(1-2): 65-80.
12. Hertog MG, Kromhout D, Aravanis C, Blackburn H, Buzina R, Fidanza F, Giampaoli S, Jansen A, Menotti A, Nedelijkovic S *et al:* "Flavonoid intake and long-term risk of coronary heart dis-ease and cancer in the seven countries study." *Arch Intern Med* 1995, 155(4): 381-386.
13. Hubbard GP, Wolffram S, Lovegrove JA, Gibbins JM: "The role of polyphenolic compounds in the diet as inhibitors of platelet function." *Proc Nutr Soc* 2003, 62(2): 469-478.
14. Wallerath T, Li H, Godtel-Ambrust U, Schwarz PM, Forstermann U: "A blend of polyphenolic compounds explains the stimulatory effect of red wine on human endothelial NO synthase." *Nitric Oxide* 2005, 12(2): 97-104.
15. Dell'Agli M, Galli GV, Vrhovsek U, Mattivi F, Bosisio E: *"In vitro* inhibition of human cGMP-specific phosphodiesterase-5 by polyphenols from red grapes." *J Agric Food Chem* 2005, 53(6): 1960-1965.
16. a) Whitley AC, Stoner GD, Darby MV, Walle T: "Intestinal epithelial cell accumulation of the cancer preventive polyphenol ellagic acid --extensive binding to protein and DNA." *Biochem Pharmacol* 2003, 66(6): 907-915.
    b) Stoner GD, Mukhtar H: "Polyphenols as cancer chemopreventive agents." *J Cell Biochem Suppl* 1995, 22: 169-180.

17. a) Dixit R, Teel RW, Daniel FB, Stoner GD: "Inhibition of benzo(a) pyrene and benzo(a)pyrene-trans- 7,8-diol metabolism and DNA binding in mouse lung explants by ellagic acid." *Cancer Res* 1985, 45(7): 2951-2956.
   b) Krichnan K, Brenner DE: "Chemoprevention of colorectal cancer." *Gastroenterol Clin North Am* 1996, 25(4): 821-858.

18. Loo G: "Redox-sensitive mechanisms of phytochemical-mediated inhibition of cancer cell proliferation" (review). *J Nutr Biochem* 2003, 14(2): 64-73.

19. Chun YJ, Kim MY, Guengerich FP, "Resveratrol is a selective human cytochrome P450 1A1 inhibitor". *Biochem Biophys Res Commun.*, 1999, 262(1): 20-24.

20. Benitez DA, Pozo-Guisado E, Alvarez-Barrientos A, Fernandez-Salguero PM, Castellon EA, "Mechanisms involved in resveratrol-induced apoptosis and cell cycle arrest in prostate cancer-derived cell lines". *Journal of Andrology* 2006, 28: 282.

21. Woo JH, Lim JH, Kim YH, Suh SI, Min do S, Chang JS, Lee YH, Park JW, Kwon TK: "Resveratrol inhibits phorbol myristate acetate-induced matrix metalloproteinase-9 expression by inhibiting JNK and PKC delta signal transduction." *Oncogene* 2004, 23(10): 1845-1853.

22. Tseng SH, Lin SM, Chen JC, Su YH, Huang HY, Chen CK, Lin PY, Chen Y: "Resveratrol suppresses the angiogenesis and tumor growth of gliomas in rats." *Clin Cancer Res* 2004, 10(6): 2190-2202.

23. Athar M, Back JH, Tang X, Kim KH, Kopelovich L, Bickers DR, Kim AL, "Resveratrol - a review of preclinical studies for human cancer prevention," *Toxicol Appl Pharmacol*, 2007, 224(3): 274-83.

24. Paliwal S, Sundaram J, Mitragotri S, "Induction of cancer-specific cytotoxcity towards human prostate and skin cells using quercetin and ultrasound," *British Journal of Cancer*, 2005, 92(3): 499-502.

25. de Sousa E, Zanatta L, Seifriz I, Creczynski-Pasa TB, Pizzolatti MG, Szpoganicz B, Silva FR: "Hypoglycemic effect and antioxidant potential of kaempferol-3, 7-O-(alpha)-dirhamnoside from Bauhinia forficata leaves." *J Nat Prod* 2004, 67(5): 829-832.

26. Kim HY, Moon BH, LeeHJ, Choi DH: "Flavonol glycosides from the leaves of Eucommia ulmoides O. with glycation inhibitory activity." *J Ethnopharmacol* 2004, 93(2-3): 227-230.

27. Kawanishi K, Ueda H, Moriyasu M: Aldose reductase inhibitors from the nature. *Curr Med Chem* 2003, 10(15): 1353-1374.

28. Lee Y: "Involvement of nuclear factor kappaB in up-regulation of aldose reductase gene expression by 12-O-tetradecanoylphorbol-13-acetate in HeLa cells." *Int J Biochem Cell Biol* 2005, Jun 1.

29, Greenspan P, Bauer JD, Pollock SH, Hargrove JL, Hartle DK: "Anti-inflammatory properties of the muscadine grape." *FASEB Journal* 2004, 18(4-5): Abst. 102.106.

30. Ref. 1, p. 80

31. ibid., p. 81

32. ibid., p. 81

33. ibid., p. 83

34. Sinclair DA: "Toward a unified theory of caloric restriction and longevity regulation." *Mech Ageing Dev* 2005, 126(9): 987-1002.

35. Joseph JA, Shukitt-Hale B, Denisova NA, Bielinkski D, Martin A, McEwen JJ, Bickford PC: "Reversals of age-related declines in neuronal signal transduction, cognitive, and motor behavioral deficits with blueberry, spinach, or strawberry dietary supplementation." *J Neurosci* 1999, 19(18): 8114-8121.

36. Moskaug JO, Carlsen H, Myhrstad M, Blomhoff R: "Polyphenols and glutathione synthesis regulation." *Am J Clin Nutr* 2005, 81(1 Suppl): 277S-283S.

37. Quideau S: "Plant 'polyphenolic' small molecules can induce a calorie restriction-mimetic lifespan extension by activating sirtuins: will 'polyphenols' someday be used as chemotherapeutic drugs in Western medicine?" *Chembiochem* 2004, 5(4): 427-430.

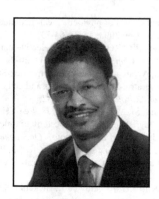

ABOUT THE AUTHOR

Dr. Allan Somersall is a practicing physician with a focus on health and wellness in the twenty-first century. He studied at the University of London, did graduate work at the University of Pennsylvania, and earned doctorate degrees in both medicine and science from the University of Toronto. He is in demand around the world for his broad range of Health Seminars to which he brings expert knowledge and contagious enthusiam. He has been a Consultant in the nutrition, health and wellness industry for over two decades and is the author of ten books.

K2 Publishing
www.muscadinepower.com
336-766-7877